The Quick Ketogenic Recipe Guide

Easy and Tasty Ketogenic Recipes to Save Your Time and Improve Your Skills

Lauren Loose

© Copyright 2021 - All rights reserved.

The content contained within this book may not be reproduced, duplicated or transmitted without direct written permission from the author or the publisher.

Under no circumstances will any blame or legal responsibility be held against the publisher, or author, for any damages, reparation, or monetary loss due to the information contained within this book. Either directly or indirectly.

Legal Notice:

This book is copyright protected. This book is only for personal use. You cannot amend, distribute, sell, use, quote or paraphrase any part, or the content within this book, without the consent of the author or publisher.

Disclaimer Notice:

Please note the information contained within this document is for educational and entertainment purposes only. All effort has been executed to present accurate, up to date, and reliable, complete information. No warranties of any kind are declared or implied. Readers acknowledge that the author is not engaging in the rendering of legal, financial, medical or professional advice. The content within this book has been derived from various sources. Please consult a licensed professional before attempting any techniques outlined in this book.

By reading this document, the reader agrees that under no circumstances is the author responsible for any losses, direct or indirect, which are incurred as a result of the use of information contained within this document, including, but not limited to, — errors, omissions, or inaccuracies.

Contents

Ketogenic Pancakes 8
Seafood Omelet 10
Salad Sandwich 12
Ground Beef and Creamy Cauliflower Made in a Skillet 13
Avocado and Salmon 16
Bacon and Eggs 17
Boiled Eggs with Mayo 18
Breakfast Salad 19
Avocado Egg Wrapped into Prosciutto 21
Cauli Flitters 23
Sheet Pan Eggs 25
Scrambled Eggs 26
Ketogenic Tapas 27
Coconut Porridge 29
Frittata with Spinach 30
Sausage Bombs 32
Pesto Bombs 33
Pork Belly Bombs 34
Cheesy Artichoke Bombs 36
Sausage and Avocado Bombs 38
Ranch and Bacon Bombs 40
Vegetable Cheese Balls 41
Chive and Blue Cheese Bombs 43
Ham and Cheese Bombs 44
Crab Rangoon Bombs 46

Brie Hazelnut Balls	48
Blue Cheese Turkey Dressed Eggs	49
Nutty Bacon Baskets	50
Crab Cakes	52
Tomato & Olive Fat Bombs	53
Creamy Olive Balls	55
Bacon Maple Pancake Balls	56
Curried Tuna Balls	57
Bacon Jalapeño Balls	58
Avocado, Macadamia, & Prosciutto Balls	59
Chocolate Cheesecake	60
Walnut Bites	63
Cinnamon Pudding	65
Cheesecake Mousse	66
No-Crust Pumpkin Pie	68
Tuscan Truffles	70
Caprese Salad Kabobs	72
Roasted Cauliflower and Tahini Yogurt Sauce	73
Zucchini Crusted Pizza	75
Stuffed Basil- Asiago Mushrooms	77
Cheese and Zucchini Roulades	79
Chicken Nuggets with Sweet Potato Crusting	81
Artichoke and Spinach Stuffed Mushrooms	83
Cobb Salad Sausage Lettuce Wraps	85
Mushroom and Asparagus Frittata	87
Sausage Balls	89

Ranch Cauliflower Crackers 91
Pork Belly Cracklings 93
Lemon Fat Bombs 94
Peanut Butter Granola 95
Grilled Turkey Burger 97
Chipotle Steak with Tortilla 99
Chicken Avocado Egg Bacon 101
Bacon Wrapped Chicken Breast 103
Avocado Pesto Pasta 105
Nutty spread Power Granola 107
Snickerdoodle Truffles 109

Ketogenic Pancakes

Preparation Time: 5 minutes

Cooking Time: 15 minutes

Servings: 4

Ingredients:

- 4 tsps. maple extract
- 8 eggs
- 4 tsps. cinnamon
- 8 coconut oil
- 2 ¾ pork rinds

Directions:

1. Put the pork in the blender and pulse until it becomes a fine powder. Then add the rest of the ingredients and mix them until smooth.
2. Heat a skillet to medium (300-400°F) and add the coconut oil into it. Pour batter into the skillet, fry it until golden brown (around 2 minutes), and of course, don't forget to flip it!
3. Bonus: If you want a sweet finish, you can add some fruit (for example strawberries) to it.

Nutrition:

2g Carbohydrates

43g Fat

24g Protein

510 Calories

Seafood Omelet

Preparation Time: 5 minutes

Cooking Time: 15 minutes

Servings: 4

Ingredients:

- 12 eggs
- 4 garlic cloves
- 1 cup mayonnaise
- 2 red chili peppers
- 10 oz. boiled shrimp or some seafood mix
- 4 tbsp. olive oil
- fennel seeds
- chives
- cumin
- 4 tbs. olive oil/butter
- salt and pepper to your taste

Directions:

1. Preheat your broiler Mix your seafood with olive oil, chili, cumin, minced garlic, salt, pepper, and fennel seeds. Then set it aside and cool to room temperature.
2. Add the chives (optional) and mayo to the cooled mixture. Whisk the eggs together, season them, and fry them in a skillet.

3. Add the mixture. When your omelet is almost ready, fold it, lower the temperature a bit, and let it set completely. Serve it immediately for the best taste.

Nutrition:

4g Carbohydrates

83g Fat

27g Protein

872 Calories

Salad Sandwich

Preparation Time: 5-10 minutes

Cooking Time: 5-10 minutes

Servings: 1

Ingredients:

- 2 oz. lettuce
- ½ avocado
- 1 cherry tomato
- 1 oz. Edam cheese (or any cheese you prefer)
- ½ oz. butter

Directions:

1. Rinse and cut the lettuce. Then use it as the base of your sandwich.
2. Cover the leaves with butter and place the cheese, avocado, and tomato on top of it.

Nutrition:

4g Carbohydrates

43g Fat

4g Protein

419 Calories

Ground Beef and Creamy Cauliflower Made in a Skillet

Preparation Time: 5 minutes

Cooking Time: 25 minutes

Servings: 4

Ingredients:

- 2 cloves garlic chopped
- 4 jalapeno peppers
- 2 tbsps. ghee
- 1 tsp. ground cumin
- 1 tsp. fish sauce
- 1 tbsp. coconut amino
- ¼ cup toasted sunflower seed oil
- ½ cup water
- 1 head cauliflower (400-500 g)
- 400-500 g lean ground beef
- 1 onion
- Salt
- Pepper
- 4 tbsps. mayo
- 4 eggs
- 1 tbsp. apple cider vinegar
- 1 tbsp. fresh parsley
- ½ ripe avocado

Directions:
1. Melt the ghee in your skillet around 300-400 °F (Medium- high). Add the onion, garlic, and jalapeno when your skillet is hot and cook it until softened (around 2-3 minutes).
2. Add the perfectly seasoned beef, keep cooking until the beef becomes completely brown. Then lower the heat to 200-300 °F (Medium-low), add the cauliflower, and continue for 2-3 minutes.
3. In the meantime, add the mayo (2 tbsp.), water, sunflower seed oil, coconut aminos, fish sauce, and cumin to a large cup and whisk them until thoroughly combined.
4. Pour it into the mixture in the skillet and stir it. Keep cooking for 3-5 minutes, until the liquids are absorbed. Remove it from the heat and spread it evenly into 4 plates.
5. Now you can crack the 4 eggs into your skillet and cook them to your liking. Meanwhile, mix 2 tbsp. mayo with your vinegar. Drizzle it over the skillet then garnish it with the diced avocado and the chopped parsley.

Nutrition:

688 Calories

52g Fat

38g Protein

14g Carbohydrates

Avocado and Salmon

Preparation Time: 5 minutes

Cooking Time: 15 minutes

Servings: 1

Ingredients:

- 1 ripe avocado
- salt
- 1 lemon (the juice part of it)
- 1 oz. goat cheese
- 2 oz. smoked salmon

Directions:

1. Cut the avocado, and remove the seed.
2. Mix the remaining ingredients, until they fuse well.
3. Place the cream inside the avocado.

Nutrition:

471 Calories

41g Fat

4g Carbs

19g Protein

Bacon and Eggs

Preparation Time: 5 minutes

Cooking Time: 10 minutes

Servings: 4

Ingredients:

- 8 eggs
- 5 oz. bacon, sliced optimal
- optional: tomatoes, parsley

Directions:

1. Cook bacon until crispy and then put it aside. Use the same pan for the eggs. Heat over a bit of medium heat and crack the eggs.
2. Cook them to your liking: repeat the same with the tomatoes, and parsley, if you are using them. Season them for your taste.
3. Tip: If you prefer it this way, you can fry the bacon and the eggs together to merge the flavors a bit better.

Nutrition:

1g Carbohydrates

22g Fat

15g Protein

272 Calories

Boiled Eggs with Mayo

Preparation Time: 3 minutes

Cooking Time: 10 minutes

Servings: 4

Ingredients:

- 8 eggs
- 8 tbsps. mayo
- avocado (optional, but recommended)

Directions:

1. Boil water in a pot, and carefully put the eggs in the water. Boil the eggs: 5-6 minutes for soft, 6-8 minutes for medium, 8-10 minutes for hard-boiled eggs.
2. Tip: Serve it with simple with the mayonnaise and the avocado. Another option is to mash together the mayo and avocado. Or you can mix everything, by smashing the eggs into the mixture and creating a delicious cream.

Nutrition:

1g Carbohydrates

29g Fat

11g Protein

316 Calories

Breakfast Salad

Preparation Time: 3 minutes

Cooking Time: 15 minutes

Servings: 2

Ingredients:

- 2 eggs
- 2 oz. avocado (sliced preferred)
- 10 grape tomatoes
- 4 strips bacon
- black pepper, salt
- 1 tsp. red wine vinegar
- 2 tsps. virgin olive oil
- 3 shredded Lacinto kale

Directions:

1. Use a bowl to combine the kale, olive oil, vinegar, and a bit of salt, and smash them with your hands until the kale softens a bit. Cook the eggs to suit your style, medium boiled recommended here, and cook your bacon.
2. Divide it into 2 plates, use your toppings, the bacon, tomatoes, and avocado for your desired outcome, and don't forget to season it.

Nutrition:

292 Calories

18g Fats
13g Carbohydrates
18g Protein

Avocado Egg Wrapped into Prosciutto

Preparation Time: 5 minutes

Cooking Time: 10 minutes

Servings: 1

Ingredients:

- 2 eggs
- 2 avocados
- 2 tsps. olive oil
- salt and pepper
- 6 prosciutto slices
- chopped parsley, tomato slices to garnish

Directions:

1. Cook the eggs for hard-boiled eggs. Cut the avocados in half, then fill the middle of them with the eggs, and cut them half too.
2. Then wrap them inside the prosciutto, and fry it over medium heat in the olive oil for roughly 10 minutes. Cook until the bacon is crispy. Drain the excess oil before serving. Use the parsley and tomato slices to make it look even better.

Nutrition:

457 Calories

33g Protein

3g Carbs
54g Fats

Cauli Flitters

Preparation Time: 10 minutes

Cooking Time: 15 minutes

Servings: 2

Ingredients:

- 2 eggs
- 1 head of cauliflower
- 1 tbsp. yeast
- sea salt, black pepper
- 1-2 tbsp. ghee
- 1 tbsp. turmeric
- 2/3 cup almond flour

Directions:

1. Put cauliflower in your pot and boil it for 8 minutes. Add the florets into a food processor and pulse them. Add the eggs, almond flour, yeast, turmeric, salt and pepper to a mixing bowl. Stir well. Form into patties.
2. Heat your ghee to medium in a skillet. Form your fritters and cook until golden on each side (3-4 minutes). Serve it while hot.

Nutrition:

238 Calories

23g Fat

5g Carbohydrates

6g Protein

Sheet Pan Eggs

Preparation Time: 5 minutes

Cooking Time: 15 minutes

Servings: 4

Ingredients:

- 12 eggs
- coconut oil
- salt and pepper to taste
- ½ cup mixed bell peppers
- ¼ cup chopped chives

Directions:

1. Preheat the oven to medium (300-400°F) Grease your baking sheet with coconut oil.
2. Mix the eggs with pepper and salt in a box until it becomes frothy, and then add the bell peppers and chopped chives.
3. Transfer mixture into the pan. Bake it for 12-15 minutes. Remove it, let it cool, and then cut it into squares.

Nutrition:

13g Protein

2g Carbs

10g Fats

507 Calories

Scrambled Eggs

Preparation Time: 2 minutes

Cooking Time: 8 minutes

Servings: 4

Ingredients:
- 4 oz. butter
- 8 eggs
- salt and pepper for taste

Directions:
1. Whisk together all the eggs, while seasoning it.
2. Melt the butter but not too brown. Transfer the eggs into the skillet and let it cook for 1-2 minutes, until they look and feel fluffy and creamy.
3. Tip: If you want to shake things up, you can pair this one up with bacon, salmon, or maybe avocado as well.

Nutrition:

1g Carbohydrates

31g Fat

11g Protein

327 Calories

Ketogenic Tapas

Preparation Time: 10 minutes

Cooking Time: 5 minutes

Servings: 4

Ingredients:

- Cheese (mozzarella, cheddar, etc.)
- Cold cuts (ham, prosciutto, salami, etc.)
- Cucumber, pepper, radishes, avocado
- mayo
- 1 lemon for its juice
- pepper, salt
- Nuts (walnuts, almonds, hazelnuts)

Direction:

1. Cut your consumables into small pieces; for example, cube with the avocado as well.
2. Mix your mayo with the lemon juice, salt, and pepper. Add the toppings as you wish
3. Tip: Use up your avocado's shell, and serve this snack in it! It will look extremely classy, trust me.

Nutrition:

5g Net Carbs

1g Fiber

57g Fat

30g protein
664 Calories

Coconut Porridge

Preparation Time: 2 minutes

Cooking Time: 10 minutes

Servings: 1

Ingredients:

- 1 egg
- 1 tbsp. coconut flour
- 1 pinch ground psyllium, husk powder
- salt
- 1 oz. butter oil/coconut oil
- 4 tbsps. coconut cream

Directions:

1. Put all ingredients to a saucepan. Mix them well and place over a low heat. Stir constantly until the desired texture.
2. Serve the mixture with coconut milk or cream. You can top it with some berries.

Nutrition:

4g Carbohydrates

49g Fat

9g Protein

486 Calories

Frittata with Spinach

Preparation Time: 5 minutes

Cooking Time: 30 minutes

Servings: 4

Ingredients:

- 8 eggs
- 8 oz. fresh spinach
- 5 oz. diced bacon
- 5 oz. shredded cheese
- 1 cup heavy whipping cream
- 2 tbsps. butter
- salt and pepper

Directions:

1. Preheat the oven to 350 °F. Cook bacon until crispy. Add the spinach and cook until wilted. Set them aside.
2. Mix cream and eggs, then pour it into the baking dish. Add the cheese, spinach, and bacon on the top, and place in the oven. Bake until golden brown for 25-30 minutes.

Nutrition:

4g Carbohydrates

59g Fat

27g Protein

661 Calories

Sausage Bombs

Preparation Time: 10 minutes

Cooking Time: 20 minutes

Servings: 20

Ingredients:

- 1 lb. Breakfast Sausage
- 1 Cup Almond Flour
- 1 Egg
- ¼ Cup Parmesan, Grated
- 1 Tablespoon Butter
- 2 Teaspoons Baking Powder

Directions:

1. Preheat your oven at 350 degree, and get a bowl. Mix all of your ingredients together before making twenty balls.
2. Place these sausage balls on a baking sheet, baking for twenty minutes. Serve warm or chilled.

Nutrition:

124 Calories

6g Protein

11g Fat

0.2g Net Carbs

Pesto Bombs

Preparation Time: 1 hour

Cooking Time: 1 hour and 5 minutes

Servings: 6

Ingredients:

- 1 Cup Cream Cheese, Full Fat
- 2 Tablespoons Basil Pesto
- 10 Green Olives, Sliced
- ½ Cup Parmesan Cheese, Grated

Directions:

1. Mix your butter and cream cheese. Mix all of your ingredients except parmesan cheese. Mix well, and then refrigerate for a half hour.
2. Roll in parmesan cheese before serving.

Nutrition:

123 Calories

4.3g Protein

12.9g Fat:

1.3g Net Carbs

Pork Belly Bombs

Preparation Time: 15 minutes

Cooking Time: 40 minutes

Servings: 6

Ingredients:

- ¼ Cup Mayonnaise
    - Ounces Pork Belly, Cooked
- 3 Bacon Slices, Cut in Half
- 1 Tablespoon Horseradish, Fresh & Grated
- 1 Tablespoon Dijon Mustard
- 6 Lettuce Leaves for Serving
- Sea Salt & Black Pepper to Taste

Directions:

1. Preheat your oven to 325, and then cook your bacon for a half hour. Allow it to cool, and then crumble your bacon. Place it in a dish.
2. Shred your pork belly, placing it in a bowl. Add in your mayonnaise, horseradish, and mustard. Mix and seasoned it.
3. Divide this mixture into six mounds, and then roll it in your crumbled bacon.
4. Serve on lettuce leaves.

Nutrition:

263 Calories

3.5g Protein

26.4g Fat

0.3g Net Carbs

Cheesy Artichoke Bombs

Preparation Time: 20 minutes

Cooking Time: 50 minutes

Servings: 4

Ingredients:

- 2 Bacon Slices
- 2 Tablespoons Ghee
- 1 Clove Garlic, Minced
- ½ Onion, Large, Peeled & Diced
- 1/3 Cup Artichoke Hearts, Canned & Sliced
- ¼ Cup Sour Cream
- 1 Tablespoon Lemon Juice, Fresh
- ¼ Cup Mayonnaise
- ¼ Cup Swiss Cheese, Grated
- 4 Avocado Halves, Pitted
- Sea Salt & Black Pepper to Taste

Directions:

1. Fry your bacon for five minutes. It should be crisp. Allow it to cool before crumbling it and placing it in a bowl. Set the bowl to the side.
2. Cook your garlic and onion in the same pan using your ghee for three minutes. Combine this in with your bacon, and then throw in your remaining ingredients.

3. Mix well, seasoning with salt and pepper. Refrigerate your mixture for a half hour before filling each avocado half with one.

Nutrition:

408 Calories

6.8g Protein

39.6g Fat

4g Net Carbs

Sausage and Avocado Bombs

Preparation Time: 20 minutes

Cooking Time: 55 minutes

Servings: 4

Ingredients:

- 12 Ounces Spanish Chorizo Sausage, Diced
- ¼ Cup Butter, Unsalted
- 2 Hardboiled Eggs, Large & Diced
- 2 Tablespoons Mayonnaise
- 2 Tablespoons Chives, Chopped
- 1 Tablespoon Lemon Juice, Fresh
- 4 Avocado Halves, Pitted
- Sea Salt to Taste
- Cayenne Pepper to Taste

Directions:

1. Fry your chorizo over heat for five minutes before placing it to the side. Get out a bowl and combine all of your ingredients, mashing it together. Make sure not to add in your avocado halves. They're for serving.
2. Refrigerate this mixture for a half hour before filling each avocado half. Serve chilled.

Nutrition:

419 Calories

11.4g Protein

38.9g Fat

2.7g Net Carbs

Ranch and Bacon Bombs

Preparation Time: 1 hour

Cooking Time: 2 hours and 30 minutes

Servings: 4

Ingredients:

- 1 Tablespoon Ranch Dressing Mix, Dry
- 8 Ounces Cream Cheese, Full Fat & Softened
- 2 Slices Bacon

Directions:

1. Preheat oven at 375 degrees, and then cook your bacon strips. They should take about fifteen minutes. Allow it to cool before crumbling it.
2. Get out a bowl and combine your cream cheese and ranch dressing mix. Stir in your bacon, and mix well. Refrigerate for two hours before serving.

Nutrition:

419 Calories

11.4g Protein

38.9g Fat

Vegetable Cheese Balls

Preparation Time: 20 minutes

Cooking Time: 55 minutes

Servings: 6

Ingredients:

- ½ Onion, Peeled & Chopped
- ½ Cup Porcini Mushrooms, Dried
- 1 Tablespoon Ghee
- ¼ Cup Butter, Unsalted
- 6 Ounces Cream Cheese, Full Fat
- 1 Clove Garlic, Chopped Fine
- 2 Cups Spinach
- Sea Salt & Black Pepper to Taste
- ¼ Cup Hard Goat Cheese, Grated

Directions:

1. Throw your butter and cream cheese in a food processor until blended well. Get a pan out and cook your garlic and onion using your ghee over medium heat. It should take three minutes, and then add in your spinach and mushrooms, cooking for another three minutes. Set it to the side so it cools.
2. Mix your butter and cream cheese with the spinach mixture, seasoning with salt and

pepper. Refrigerate it for a half hour, and make it into five hours. Roll it into your goat cheese before serving.

Nutrition:

166 Calories

3.4g Protein

16.7g Fat

Chive and Blue Cheese Bombs

Preparation Time: 15 minutes

Cooking Time: 45 minutes

Servings: 6

Ingredients:

- ¼ Cup Butter, Unsalted
- ½ Cup Blue Cheese, Crumbled
    - Ounces Cream Cheese, Full Fat
- 2 Spring Onions, Chopped
- 1/3 Cup Chives, Fresh & Chopped
- 1 Tablespoon Parsley, Chopped

Directions:

1. Throw your butter and cream cheese in a food processor, mixing until well blended. Add in all of your remaining ingredients except for chives, making sure it's mixed well. Chill mixture for a half hour, and roll in chives before serving.

Nutrition:

157 Calories

5g Protein

16.2g Fat

Ham and Cheese Bombs

Preparation Time: 20 minutes

Cooking Time: 45 minutes

Servings: 6

Ingredients:

- ¼ Cup Butter, Unsalted
- ¼ Cup Cheddar Cheese, Grated
- 12 Ounces Cream Cheese, Full Fat
- 2 Tablespoons Basil, Fresh & Chopped
- 6 Slices Parma Ham
- 6 Green Olives, Large & Pitted
- Black Pepper to Taste

Directions:

1. Use a food processor to blend your butter and cream cheese together. Add your basil and cheddar cheese, mixing well season with black pepper, and then place it in the fridge for a half hour. Make six balls from your mixture, and then roll each one in Parma ham, topping with an olive to serve. You'll need a toothpick to hold the olive in place.

Nutrition:

167 Calories

6.4g Protein

16.7g Fat

Crab Rangoon Bombs

Preparation Time: 20 minutes

Cooking Time: 40 minutes

Servings: 12

Ingredients:

- 8 Ounces Cream Cheese
- 1 Can Crab
- ½ Teaspoon Garlic Powder
- ½ Teaspoon Onion Powder
- ½ Teaspoon Garlic, Minced
- ¾ Cup Mozzarella Cheese, Shredded
- 10 Slices Bacon
- Sea Salt & Black Pepper to Taste

Directions:

1. Heat your oven to 325, and then get out a baking sheet. Line it with parchment paper, and then bake for thirty minutes. Allow your bacon to cool before you crumble it. Set it to the side, and then mix all of your remaining ingredients in a bowl.
2. Let it rest and roll twenty-four balls. Roll them in your crumbled bacon before serving.

Nutrition:

227 Calories

13.8g Protein

2.1g Fat

Brie Hazelnut Balls

Preparation Time: 2 hours 5 minutes

Cooking Time: 20 minutes

Servings: 6

Ingredients:

- 4 oz. Brie
- 2 oz. hazelnuts, toasted
- 1/8 tsp. fresh thyme, finely chopped

Directions:

1. Combine all ingredients until coarse, doughy mixture is formed, about 30 seconds. Scrape mixture and transfer to a bowl, then refrigerate 2 hours. Form into 6 balls. Serve or refrigerate up to 3 days.

Nutrition:

2g Total Carbohydrates

11g Fat

5g Protein

121 Calories

Blue Cheese Turkey Dressed Eggs

Preparation Time: 1 hour 20 minutes

Cooking Time: 12 minutes

Servings: 6

Ingredients:

- 6 hard-boiled eggs
- 2 green onions
- 6 oz. smoked turkey breast, chopped
- ½ cup blue cheese, crumbled
- 2 tbsp. Blue cheese dressing
- ¼ cup mayonnaise
- 2 tbsp. hot mustard
- ½ rib celery

Directions:

1. Chop the turkey and celery. Take the egg yolks out and cut in half. Mix remaining ingredients except for green onions. Grate the green onions over the mixture. Mix all ingredients together. With the teaspoon fill egg halves with the mixture. Refrigerate for one hour. Serve.

Nutrition:

11.5 g Fat

14 g Protein

167 Calories

Nutty Bacon Baskets

Preparation Time: 15 minutes

Cooking Time: 20 minutes

Servings: 6

Ingredients:

- 12 slices bacon, 6 cuts in half
- 4 slices cooked bacon, chopped into bits
- 1 Tbsp. butter
- ½ cup pecans
- ½ cup macadamia nuts
- ¼ tsp. granulated garlic
- 1/8 tsp. freshly ground black pepper

Directions:

1. Preheat oven to 400°F. Put half-strip bacon in an X shape in the bottom of 6 cups. Put 1 full slice bacon along with the inside of the cup vertically.
2. Put cookie sheet under the cups and bake until slightly browned and crisp. Meanwhile, melt butter. Mix in nuts, garlic, and pepper and cook 4-5 minutes. Remove from heat.
3. Once cooled, coarsely chop nut mixture and combine with bacon bits. Divide nut mixture between cups and serve.

Nutrition:

44 g Fat

9 g Protein

437 Calories

Crab Cakes

Preparation Time: 40 minutes

Cooking Time: 30 minutes

Servings: 4

Ingredients:

- 1 lb. crabmeat
- 1 egg
- 1 tbsp. Worcestershire sauce
- 1 tbsp. mayonnaise
- 1 tbsp. parsley
- Salt to taste

Directions:

1. In a bowl mix together egg, Worcester-shire sauce, mayonnaise, parsley and season with salt. Add in crabmeat, mix and form into cakes. Place onto a baking sheet lined up with parchment paper. Refrigerate for 30 minutes. Bake for 30 minutes or until heated through at 375°F.

Nutrition:

10 g Fat

19 g Protein

203 Calories

Tomato & Olive Fat Bombs

Preparation Time: 45 minutes

Cooking Time: 10 minutes

Servings: 6

Ingredients:

- 3½ oz. full-fat cream cheese
- ¼ cup unsalted butter
- ¼ cup Manchego cheese, grated
- ¼ cup sun-dried tomatoes, drained, chopped
- ¼ cup green olives, pitted, sliced
- 2 tbsp. capers, drained
- 1 garlic clove, crushed
- 1/3 cup flaked almonds, raw or toasted
- Pepper to taste

Directions:

1. Mix butter and cream cheeses until smooth. Add the next five ingredients. Season with pepper. Mix well. Refrigerate for 30 minutes. Make 6 balls out of the mixture. Roll each ball in the almond flakes. Serve.

Nutrition:

18.1 g Fat

4.2 g Protein

178 Calories

Creamy Olive Balls

Preparation Time: 40 minutes

Cooking Time: 10 minutes

Servings: 6

Ingredients:

- 6 large kalamata olives, pitted
- 2 tbsp. cream cheese
- 1 tbsp. coconut oil, melted
- 2 tbsp. hemp hearts

Directions:

1. Blend olives, cream cheese, and coconut oil until well mixed. Refrigerate mixture for 30 minutes, or until it solidifies. Once the mixture is solid, remove from refrigerator and shape into 6 balls. Place the plate and roll balls to coat.

Nutrition:

Fat 4 g

Protein 3 g

Calories 71

Bacon Maple Pancake Balls

Preparation Time: 10 minutes

Cooking Time: 10 minutes

Servings: 6

Ingredients:

- 3 oz. bacon, cooked
- 3 oz. cream cheese
- ½ tsp. maple flavor
- ¼ tsp. salt
- 3 tbsp. crushed pecans

Directions:

1. Chop bacon into small pieces. In a bowl, combine cream cheese and bacon with maple flavor and salt. Mix well with a fork. Form mixture into 6 balls. Put crushed pecans on a plate and roll into balls to coat evenly.

Nutrition:

1g Total Carbs

13g Fat

6g Protein

148 Calories

Curried Tuna Balls

Preparation Time: 10 minutes

Cooking Time: 10 minutes

Servings: 6

Ingredients:

- 3 oz. tuna in oil, drained
- 2 oz. cream cheese
- ¼ tsp. curry powder, divided
- 1 oz. crumbled macadamia nuts

Directions:

1. In a small food processor, mix tuna, cream cheese, and half the curry powder until smooth, about 30 seconds. Form mixture into 6 balls. Mix macadamia nuts and curry powder then roll individual balls through to coat evenly.

Nutrition:

1g Total Carbs

8g Fat

5g Protein

93 Calories

Bacon Jalapeño Balls

Preparation Time: 10 minutes

Cooking Time: 10 minutes

Servings: 6

Ingredients:

- 3 oz. bacon, cooked, fat reserved
- 3 oz. cream cheese
- 2 tbsp. bacon fat, reserved
- 1 tsp. jalapeño pepper, seeded, finely chopped
- 1 tbsp. cilantro, finely chopped

Directions:

1. Cut bacon into tiny pieces. In a bowl, combine cream cheese, bacon fat, jalapeño, and cilantro. Mix well with a fork. Form mixture into 6 balls. Place bacon pieces on a medium plate and roll individual balls through to coat evenly.

Nutrition:

11g Fat

7g Protein

135 Calories

Avocado, Macadamia, & Prosciutto Balls

Preparation Time: 7 minutes

Cooking Time: 10 minutes

Servings: 6

Ingredients:

- 4 oz. macadamia nuts
- 4 oz. avocado pulp
- 1 oz. cooked prosciutto, crumbled
- ¼ tsp. freshly ground black pepper

Directions:

1. Blend macadamia nuts until evenly crumbled. Slip it into half. Mix avocado, half the macadamia nuts, prosciutto, and pepper. Mix well with a fork. Form mixture into 6 balls. Place remaining crumbled macadamia nuts on a medium plate and roll individual balls through to coat evenly. Serve immediately.

Nutrition:

17g Fat

3g Protein

170 Calories

Chocolate Cheesecake

Preparation Time: 10 minutes

Cooking Time: 2 hours

Servings: 12

Ingredients

- 1/4 cup almond flour
- 1/4 cup cocoa powder
- 1/4 cup Swerve sweetener
- 3 tablespoons melted vegan butter
- 6 ounces' dark chocolate
- 1 tablespoon vegan butter
- 24 ounces cream cheese
- 1/2 cup Swerve sweetener
- Sweetener with 1 cup of powder
- 1 tablespoon vanilla extract
- 3 large eggs
- 1/4 cup cocoa powder
- 1/3 cup thick cream
- 2 teaspoons melted butter
- 3/4 fresh cane
- 3 oz. chopped chocolate
- 1/2 teaspoon vanilla extract

Direction:

1. Preheat oven to 325F. Mix the almond flour, cocoa powder, and sweetener. Stir in the melted butter.
2. Press the mixture well into the bottom of a 9-inch bow-shaped container. Bake 10 minutes, then remove and reduce oven temperature to 300F.
3. In a small saucepan over medium heat, mix the dark chocolate with butter. Set aside.
4. Beat cream cheese, sweeteners and vanilla extract, then eggs one by one, scraping the sides and sides of the bowl.
5. Mix cocoa powder and thick cream, then add melted chocolate.
6. Grease with melted butter, don't disturb the crust. Put filling into the pan and shake gently.
7. Bake 60 minutes. Remove and let cool completely. After cooling, remove the sides, cover well in a plastic wrap and refrigerate for at least 3 hours.
8. Over medium heat, incorporate cream and the sweetener. Simmer, put off heat and add chopped chocolate and vanilla. Set aside and then beat until smooth.

9. Pour over the top of cold cheese.

Nutrition

32.98g fat

7.75g protein

5.22g carbohydrates

Walnut Bites

Preparation Time: 15 minutes

Cooking Time: 0 minute

Serving: 16

Ingredients

- 1 ½ cup Old Fashioned oats
- 3 tablespoons dark cocoa
- ½ teaspoon cinnamon
- 1 cup pitted soft dates
- 3 tablespoons almond butter
- 3 tablespoons dark pure maple syrup
- 3 tablespoons chopped walnuts
- 3 tablespoons mini chocolate chips

Direction:

1. Crush the oatmeal. Transfer in bowl. Mix cocoa, cinnamon and salt.
2. Crush dates then add almond butter and maple syrup to make a thick paste.
3. Mold the dough to the silicone to begin to resemble crushed cookie dough, about 2 minutes. Continue the work on the dough. Mix nuts and chocolate chips.
4. Knead well. Form into 14 balls. Refrigerate the refrigerator to adjust the chocolate.

Nutrition

4g Fat

5g Carbohydrates

2g Protein

Cinnamon Pudding

Preparation Time: 10 minutes

Cooking Time: 1 hour

Servings: 6

Ingredients

- 3 eggs
- 3/4 cup thick cream
- 1/2 splendid cane
- 1/4 cup unsweetened caramel topping
- 1 cup almond flour
- 1/4 teaspoon baking powder
- 1 cup cottage cheese
- 1/4 teaspoon cinnamon

Direction:

1. Beat all the ingredients with the mixer
2. Pour into an 8x8 "glass baking dish with butter and sprinkle extra cinnamon.
3. Bake at 350 ° F for 1 hour.

Nutrition

18g fat

2g protein

8g carbohydrates

Cheesecake Mousse

Preparation Time: 5 minutes

Cooking Time: 0 minutes

Servings: 6

Ingredients

- 8 ounces softened cream cheese
- 1/3 cup erythritol powder
- 1/8 teaspoon concentrated stevia powder
- 1 1/2 teaspoons vanilla extract
- 1/4 teaspoon lemon extract
- 1 cup thick whipped cream

Direction:

1. Beat the cream cheese until smooth.
2. Mix the extract of erythritol, stevia, vanilla, and lemon.
3. Beat the thick cream with the mixer until stiff peaks form.
4. Fold half the whisk in the cream cheese mixture. Fold the other half of the whip.
5. Beat until it is soft and fluffy.
6. In the refrigerator for 2 hours. Melt with fresh fruit.

Nutrition

27.8g fat

3.7g protein

16.5 g carbohydrates

No-Crust Pumpkin Pie

Preparation Time: 10 minutes

Cooking Time: 40 minutes

Servings: 10

Ingredients

- 2 tablespoons butter
- 4 tablespoons coconut without sugar
- 15 oz. pumpkin
- 2/3 heavy fresh cane
- 1-ounce butter
- 2 teaspoons pumpkin pie
- 1 teaspoon baking powder
- 3 eggs
- 1/4 cups thick cream

Direction:

1. Chop squash into cubes and position it in a pan. Boil wheat, butter and salt over medium heat.
2. Simmer for 20 minutes. Stir occasionally.
3. Once it soft, mix the remaining ingredients, except the eggs with a hand blender.
4. Whisk eggs with a hand mixer for 3 minutes. Add the purified pumpkin and mix.

5. Prep oven to 400 ° F. Grease a 9 "baking dish with butter and apply the coconut flakes evenly.
6. Bake for 20 minutes.

Nutrition

10g fat

2g protein

2g carbohydrates

Tuscan Truffles

Preparation Time: 10 minutes

Cooking Time: 25 minutes

Serving: 6

Ingredients

- 2 logs of goat cheese
- 8 ounces of mascarpone cheese
- 6 tbsps. of parmesan cheese (grated)
- 3 cloves of garlic (minced)
- 2 tsps. of olive oil
- 1 tsp. of white balsamic vinegar
- 3/4 tsp. of lemon zest (grated)
- 6 ½ tbsp. of prosciutto (chopped)
- 5 tbsps. of dried figs (chopped)
- 3 tbsps. of parsley (minced)
- ¼ tsp. of pepper
- 1 cup of pine nuts (chopped)

Directions:

1. Mix the first eleven listed ingredients in a large bowl. Shape the mixture into thirty-six small balls. Roll the balls in chopped pine nuts. Refrigerate for twenty minutes.

Nutrition:

82.3 Calories

3.3g Protein

7.3g Fat

Caprese Salad Kabobs

Preparation Time: 10 minutes

Cooking Time: 10 minutes

Servings: 4 servings

Ingredients
- 24 grape tomatoes
- 12 small bits of mozzarella cheese balls
- 24 basil leaves.
- 3 tbsps. of olive oil
- 2 tsps. of balsamic vinegar

Directions:
1. Combine vinegar along with olive oil in a small bowl. Thread two tomatoes, two leaves of basil, and one ball of cheese alternately on each skewer. Drizzle the mixture of olive oil over the skewers. Serve immediately.

Nutrition:

45.4 Calories

2.3g Protein

1.6g Carbs

Roasted Cauliflower and Tahini Yogurt Sauce

Preparation Time: 10 minutes

Cooking Time: 55 minutes

Serving: 4

Ingredients

- ¼ cup of parmesan cheese (grated)
- 3 tbsps. of olive oil
- 2 cloves of garlic (minced)
- ¼ tsp. of salt
- 1/3 tsp. of pepper
- 1 cauliflower (cut in four wedges)

For the sauce:

- ½ cup of Greek yogurt
- 1 tbsp. of lemon juice
- ½ tbsp. of tahini
- ¼ tsp. of salt
- 1 pinch of paprika
- Parsley (minced)

Directions:

1. Preheat your oven at one hundred and fifty degrees Celsius. Mix the first five ingredients. Rub the mixture over the wedges of cauliflower. Grease a baking tray with cooking spray.

2. Arrange the wedges of cauliflower on the baking tray. Roast for forty minutes. For the sauce, combine lemon juice, yogurt, seasonings, and tahini in a bowl. Serve the cauliflower wedges and drizzle tahini sauce on top. Garnish with parsley.

Nutrition:

179.6 Calories

7.6g Protein

15.4g Fat

Zucchini Crusted Pizza

Preparation Time: 10 minutes

Cooking Time: 45 minutes

Serving: 6

Ingredients

- 2 large eggs (beaten)
- 2 cups of zucchini (shredded, squeezed)
- ½ cup of mozzarella cheese (shredded)
- 1/3 cup of parmesan cheese (grated)
- ¼ cup of flour
- 1 tbsp. of olive oil
- 1 ½ tbsp. of basil (minced)
- 1 tsp. of thyme (minced)

For the toppings:

- 12 ounces of sweet red pepper (roasted, julienned)
- 1 cup of mozzarella cheese (shredded)
- ½ cup of turkey pepperoni (sliced)

Directions:

1. Preheat your oven at two hundred degrees Celsius. Combine the first eight listed ingredients in a bowl. Transfer the mixture to a greased pizza pan. Spread the mixture and evenly press it to the base.

2. Bake for sixteen minutes. Add the toppings on the pizza. Bake for twelve minutes. Slice the pizza using a pizza cutter. Serve hot.

Nutrition:

226.3 Calories

13.6g Protein

8.6g Carbs

Stuffed Basil- Asiago Mushrooms

Preparation Time: 10 minutes

Cooking Time: 35 minutes

Serving: 4

Ingredients

- 24 Portobello mushrooms (remove the stems)
- ½ cup of mayonnaise
- ¾ cup of Asiago cheese(shredded)
- 1/3 cup of basil leaves (remove the stems)
- ¼ tsp. of white pepper
- 12 cherry tomatoes (halved)

Directions:

1. Preheat your oven at one hundred and fifty degrees Celsius. Grease a baking dish with cooking spray. Arrange the mushroom caps in the dish. Bake the mushrooms for ten minutes.
2. Combine Asiago cheese, mayonnaise, pepper, and basil in a food processor. Mix well. Fill the mushroom caps with the cheese and basil mixture. Top each mushroom cap with half a tomato.
3. Bake for ten minutes. Serve warm.

Nutrition:

36.6 Calories

2.3g Protein
3.3g Fat

Cheese and Zucchini Roulades

Preparation Time: 10 minutes

Cooking Time: 25 minutes

Serving: 6

Ingredients

- 1 cup of ricotta cheese
- ¼ cup of parmesan cheese (grated)
- 2 tbsps. of basil (minced)
- 1 tbsp. of capers
- 1 ½ tbsp. of Greek olives (chopped)
- 1 tsp. of lemon zest (grated)
- 2 tbsps. of lemon juice
- 1/8 tsp. of pepper
- 1/4 tsp. of salt
- 4 zucchinis

Directions:

1. Combine the first nine listed ingredients in a bowl. Slice the zucchinis into twenty-four slices lengthwise. Grease a grill rack with cooking spray. Cook the slices of zucchini for three minutes.
2. Add one tbsp. of the ricotta cheese mixture on one end of the zucchini slices. Roll up the slices. Secure using toothpicks. Serve immediately.

Nutrition:

29.4 Calories

3.5g Protein

1.6g Fat

Chicken Nuggets with Sweet Potato Crusting

Preparation Time: 10 minutes

Cooking Time: 30 minutes

Serving: 4

Ingredients

- 1 cup of sweet potato chips
- ¼ cup of flour
- 1 tsp. of salt
- ½ tsp. of ground pepper (ground)
- ¼ tsp. of baking powder
- 1 tbsp. of cornstarch
- 1 pound of chicken tenderloins (cut in pieces of half-inch)
- Oil (to fry)

Directions:

1. Heat the oil in a large skillet. Add flour, chips, salt, baking powder, and pepper in a food processor. Pulse the ingredients for making a ground mixture.
2. Toss the chicken pieces in cornstarch. Shake off excess cornstarch. Toss in the chip mixture. Press the chicken pieces gently for coating. Fry

the chicken nuggets for three minutes. Serve hot.

Nutrition:

305.6 Calories

26.6g Protein

18.9g Fat

Artichoke and Spinach Stuffed Mushrooms

Preparation Time: 10 minutes

Cooking Time: 40 minutes

Servings: 6

Ingredients

- 3 ounces of cream cheese
- ½ cup of mayonnaise
- 1 cup of sour cream
- ¾ tsp. of garlic salt
- 1 can of artichoke hearts (chopped)
- 10 ounces of spinach (chopped)
- 1/3 cup of mozzarella cheese (shredded)
- 3 tbsps. of parmesan cheese (shredded)
- 30 large mushrooms (remove the stems)

Directions:

1. Preheat your oven at two hundred degrees Celsius. Combine the first four listed ingredients in a bowl. Add spinach, artichoke, three tbsps. Of parmesan cheese, and mozzarella cheese.
2. Arrange the mushrooms on a large aluminum foil-lined baking tray. Add one tbsp. of the filling into the mushroom caps. Sprinkle

remaining parmesan cheese from the top. Bake for twenty minutes.

Nutrition:

52.2 Calories

2.6g Protein

5.6g Fat

Cobb Salad Sausage Lettuce Wraps

Preparation Time: 10 minutes

Cooking Time: 25 minutes

Servings: 6

Ingredients

- 3/4 cup of ranch salad dressing
- 1/3 cup of blue cheese (crumbled)
- 1/4 cup of watercress (chopped)
- 1 pound of pork sausage
- 2 tbsps. of chives (minced)
- 6 leaves of iceberg lettuce
- 1 avocado (peeled, diced)
- 4 boiled eggs (chopped)
- 1 tomato (chopped)

Directions

1. Combine blue cheese, dressing, and watercress in a bowl. Heat some oil in an iron skillet. Add the sausage. Cook for seven minutes and crumble. Add the chives.
2. Spoon the sausage mixture into the leaves of lettuce. Top the sausage mixture with eggs, tomato, and avocado. Drizzle the mixture of dressing on top. Serve immediately.

Nutrition:

430.6 Calories

16.5g Protein

39.6g Fat

Mushroom and Asparagus Frittata

Preparation Time: 10 minutes

Cooking Time: 45 minutes

Serving: 8

Ingredients

- 8 large eggs
- 1/2 cup of ricotta cheese
- 2 tbsps. of lemon juice
- 1/2 tsp. of salt
- 1/4 tsp. of pepper
- 1 tbsp. of olive oil
- 8 ounces of asparagus spears
- 1 onion (sliced)
- 1/3 cup of sweet green pepper
- 3/4 cup of Portobello mushrooms (sliced)

Directions:

1. Preheat your oven at one hundred and fifty degrees Celsius. Combine ricotta cheese, eggs, pepper, lemon juice, and salt in a bowl. Heat oil in an iron skillet. Add onion, asparagus, mushrooms, and red pepper. Cook for eight minutes. Remove the asparagus from the skillet.

2. Cut the spears of asparagus into pieces of two-inch. Return the spears to the skillet. Add the mixture of eggs. Bake in the oven for twenty minutes. Let the frittata sit for five minutes.
3. Cut the frittata into wedges. Serve warm.

Nutrition:

132.2 Calories

9.3g Protein

8.2g Fat

Sausage Balls

Preparation Time: 10 minutes

Cooking Time: 45 minutes

Servings: 6

Ingredients

- 1 pound of spicy pork sausage (ground)
- 8 ounces of cream cheese
- 1/2 cup of cheddar cheese (shredded)
- 1/3 cup of parmesan cheese (shredded)
- 1 tbsp. of Dijon mustard
- 1/2 tsp. of garlic powder
- 1/4 tsp. of salt

Directions:

1. Preheat your oven at one hundred and seventy degrees Celsius. Use parchment paper for lining a baking sheet. Combine cream cheese, sausage, parmesan cheese, cheddar cheese, garlic powder, mustard, and salt in a mixing bowl. Mix well.
2. Take one tbsp. of the mixture. Roll it into a ball. Repeat for the remaining mixture. Arrange the prepared balls on the lined baking tray. Bake for thirty minutes. Serve hot.

Nutrition:

102.3 Calories
5.9g Protein
9.6g Fat

Ranch Cauliflower Crackers

Preparation Time: 10 minutes

Cooking Time: 70 minutes

Serving: 6

Ingredients

- 12 ounces of cauliflower rice
- Cheesecloth
- 1 large egg
- 1 tbsp. of ranch salad dressing mix (dry)
- 1/8 tsp. of cayenne pepper
- 1 cup of parmesan cheese (shredded)

Directions:

1. Add the cauliflower rice in a large bowl. Microwave for four minutes covered. Transfer the cauliflower rice to a strainer lined with cheesecloth. Squeeze out excess moisture. Preheat oven at two hundred degrees Celsius. Use parchment paper for lining a baking tray.
2. Combine egg, cauliflower rice, ranch mix, and pepper in a bowl. Add the cheese. Mix well. Take two tbsps. Of the mixture and add them to the baking tray. Flatten with your hands. The thinner you can make the mixture; the crispier will be the crackers.

3. Bake for ten minutes. Flip the crackers. Bake for ten minutes. Serve warm.

Nutrition:

29.6 Calories

2.6g Protein

2.6g Fat

Pork Belly Cracklings

Preparation Time: 10 minutes

Cooking Time: 80 minutes

Serving: 6

Ingredients

- 3 pounds of pork belly (with skin)
- 2 cups of water
- 4 tbsps. of Cajun seasoning

Directions:

1. Keep the pork belly in the refrigerator for forty minutes. Cut the pork into cubes of three-fourth inch. Fill a cast-iron pot with one-fourth portion of water. Add one tsp. of Cajun seasoning. Boil the water.
2. Add the cubes of pork belly. Cook for twenty minutes. Cover the pot once fat begins to pop and sizzle. Cook for fifteen minutes. Drain the pork cracklings.
3. Sprinkle remaining seasoning from the top. Serve immediately.

Nutrition:

210.3 Calories

16.5g Protein

16.6g Fat

Lemon Fat Bombs

Preparation Time: 10 minutes

Cooking Time: 50 minutes

Serving: 4

Ingredients

- 1 cup of shredded coconut (dry)
- 1/4 cup of coconut oil
- 3 tbsps. of erythritol sweetener (powdered)
- 1 tbsps. of lemon zest
- 1 pinch of salt

Directions:

1. Add the coconut in a high-power blender. Blend until creamy for fifteen minutes. Add sweetener, coconut oil, salt, and lemon zest. Blend for two minutes. Fill small muffin cups with the coconut mixture. Chill in the refrigerator for thirty minutes.

Nutrition:

69.9 Calories

0.5g Protein

7.9g Fat

Peanut Butter Granola

Preparation Time: 10 minutes

Cooking Time: 40 minutes

Servings: 12

Ingredients

- 2 cups Almonds
- 2 cups Pecans
- 1 cup of shredded coconut
- ¼ cup Sunflower seeds
- ¼ cup Water
- ¼ cup Butter
- 1/3 cup Sweetener
- 1/3 cup Vanilla protein powder
- 1/3 cup Peanut butter

Directions:

1. Preheat your oven at one hundred and fifty degrees Celsius. Use parchment paper for lining a large baking tray. Add pecans and almonds in a blender. Process for two minutes.
2. Combine processed mixture with sweetener, coconut, vanilla protein powder, and sunflower seeds. Melt butter along with peanut butter in a bowl. Add melted butter mixture over the mixture of nuts. Mix well. Spread the nut

mixture on the baking tray evenly. Bake for thirty minutes.

Nutrition:

335.9 Calories

10.6g Protein

31.2g Fat

Grilled Turkey Burger

Preparation Time: 5 minutes

Cooking Time: 10 minutes

Servings: 4

Ingredients

- 1 lb. ground turkey breasts
- 1/2 cup almond flour
- 1 large egg
- 1/4 cup yellow onion
- 1/4 cup chopped parsley
- 1 clove minced garlic
- 1 tbsp. extra virgin olive oil
- Salt and pepper to taste

Directions

1. In a bowl, mix turkey, egg, almond flour, parsley, garlic and onions. Season it, and then mix them all well. Evenly shape the mixture into four identical patties. Use extra virgin olive oil with brush on both sides.

2. Add some oil to a non-stick grilling pan on medium-high heat. Now, place the patties you made on the grill and cook for about five to six minutes. Turn the patties and cook for another

five to six minutes. Finally, wrap the patties in a lettuce and eat away!

Nutrition:

340 Calories

21g Fat

2.5g Fiber

Chipotle Steak with Tortilla

Preparation Time: 5 minutes

Cooking Time: 15 minutes

Servings: 4

Ingredients

- 16 oz. skirt steak
- 4 oz. pepper jack cheese
- 1 cup sour cream
- 1 handful fresh cilantro
- 1 tbsp. extra virgin olive oil
- 1 splash chipotle tabasco sauce
- Salt and pepper to taste

Homemade Guacamole

- 2 avocado(s)
- 2 tsp. lime juice
- 2 tbsp. fresh cilantro
- Salt and pepper to taste

Directions

1. Season your skirt steak to taste with salt and pepper. Then, on high heat, heat a cast iron skillet. Add olive oil when the skillet is hot and cook the skirt steak for around four minutes on each side.

2. Place it on a plate to rest while you prepare the guacamole. Slice the steak against the grain and make it into bite-sized strips. Divide the same into four equal portions.
3. Add the cheese to the top portion. Follow that with ¼ cup of guacamole and ¼ cup of sour cream. Splash each portion with some chipotle tabasco sauce (not necessary) and fresh cilantro.
4. Prepare the guacamole and serve with low carb tortillas. For homemade guacamole, remove the pit from the avocado and then mash the content. Add the rest of the ingredients and serve.

Nutrition:

810 Calories

61g Fat

15g Carbohydrates

Chicken Avocado Egg Bacon

Preparation Time: 10 minutes

Cooking Time: 10 minutes

Servings: 4

Ingredients

- 12 oz. cooked chicken breast
- 6 slices crumbled bacon
- 3 boiled eggs cut into cubes
- 1 cup cherry tomatoes cut into halves
- 1/2 small sliced red onion
- 1 large avocado(s)
- 1/2 stick finely chopped celery

Salad Dressing

- 1/2 cup olive oil mayonnaise
- 2 tbsp. sour cream
- 1 tsp. Dijon mustard
- 4 tbsp. extra virgin olive oil
- 2 cloves minced garlic
- 2 tsp. lemon juice
- 4 cups lettuce
- Salt and pepper to taste

Directions

1. Combine all the ingredients together and mix them well for the salad dressing. Then, combine

chicken, tomatoes, bacon, eggs, red onions, and celery together. Add about ¾ of the salad dressing and mix them well.
2. Add the avocado and toss together gently. Check the taste and, if needed, add the remainder of the salad dressing as well. Finally, add salt and pepper to taste and then serve it over lettuce.

Nutrition:

387 Calories

27g Fat

2.5g Carbohydrates

Bacon Wrapped Chicken Breast

Preparation Time: 10 minutes

Cooking Time: 45 minutes

Servings: 4

Ingredients

- 4 boneless, skinless chicken breasts
- 8 oz. sharp cheddar cheese
- 8 slices bacon
- 4 oz. sliced jalapeno peppers
- 1 tsp. garlic powder
- Salt and pepper to taste

Directions

1. Preheat the oven at around 3500F. Ensure to season both sides of chicken breast well with salt, garlic powder, and pepper. Place the chicken breast on a non-stick baking sheet (foil-covered). Cover the chicken with cheese and add jalapeno slices. Cut the bacon slices in half and then place the four halves over each piece of chicken. Bake for around 30 to 45 minutes at most. If the chicken is set but the bacon still feels undercooked, you may want to put it under the broiler for a few minutes. Once

done, serve hot with a side of low carb garlic parmesan roasted asparagus.

Nutrition:

640 Calories

48g Fat

6g Carbohydrates

Avocado Pesto Pasta

Preparation Time: 5 minutes

Cooking Time: 10 minutes

Servings: 2

Ingredients

- 4 oz. boneless chicken thighs
- 2 zucchinis
- 4 tbsp. extra virgin olive oil
- 1 tbsp. coconut oil
- 1 avocado
- 1/2 cup water
- 1/2 cup fresh basil
- 1 clove minced garlic
- Salt and pepper to taste

Directions

1. In a non-stick pan, heat the coconut oil on medium heat. Add the chicken after the oil has melted and cook until the chicken is no longer pink in color.
2. Use a spiralizer while the chicken is cooking and make zoodles out of the zucchinis. Add these to a non-stick pan and cook for around five minutes. Add all other ingredients together in a blender until the mixture is smooth.

3. Add everything to a bowl once the chicken is done. Mix them well so that the avocado sauce we made covers the entire zucchini noodles. Serve them warm and enjoy a scrumptious one!

Nutrition:

440 Calories

40g Fat

16g Carbohydrates

Nutty spread Power Granola

Preparation time: 10 minutes

Cooking time: 5 minutes

Servings: 12 servings

Ingredients:

1 1/2 cups of almonds

1 1/2 cups of walnuts

1 cup destroyed coconut or almond flour.

1/4 cup of sunflower seeds

1/3 cup of Swerve Sweetener

1/3 cup of vanilla whey protein powder

1/3 cup of nutty spread

1/4 cup of margarine

1/4 cup of water

Directions:

Preheat broiler to 300F and line a huge, rimmed heating sheet with a paper material.

In a food processor, process almonds and walnuts until they look like coarse scraps with some bigger parts. Move to a large bowl and mix with destroyed coconut, sunflower seeds, sugar, and vanilla protein powder.

In a microwave-safe bowl, soften the nutty spread and margarine together.

Pour softened nutty spread blend over nut blend and mix well, stirring gently. Mix in water. Blend will cluster together.

Spread blend evenly on a prepared sheet and heat for 30 minutes. Take it out and let it cool.

Nutrition:

Calories: 338 kcal

Total Fat: 17g

Saturated Fat: 3.5g

Sodium: 80mg

Total Carbohydrates: 60g

Fiber: 8g

Total Sugars: 14g

Snickerdoodle Truffles

Preparation time: 10 minutes

Cooking time: 10 minutes

Servings: 4 servings

Ingredients:

2 cups of almond flour

1/2 cup of Swerve, Confectioners

1 tsp. of cream of tartar

1 tsp. of ground cinnamon

1/4 tsp. of salt

6 tbsps. Spread, softened.

1 tsp. of vanilla concentrate

3 tbsps. Swerve, Granular

1 tsp. of ground cinnamon

Directions:

In a large bowl, whisk together the almond flour, Swerve, cream of tartar, cinnamon, and salt. Mix in dissolved spread and vanilla concentrate until the batter meets up. If the mixture is too brittle to even think about squeezing together, add a tablespoon of water and mix.

Scoop mixture out by the adjusted tablespoon and crush in your palm a couple of times to help in binding, at that point fold into a ball. Spot on a waxed paper sheet and rehash with residual batter.

In a shallow bowl, whisk together the Swerve and the cinnamon. Roll the truffles in the covering until all around secured.

Nutrition:

Calories: 121

Total Fat: 8.9g

Cholesterol: 0mg

Sodium: 201mg

Total Carbs: 5.8g

Fiber: 2.4g

Sugars: 0.2g

Protein: 4g

www.ingramcontent.com/pod-product-compliance
Lightning Source LLC
Chambersburg PA
CBHW070722030426
42336CB00013B/1897